BODY TALK
NEVER
LIES...

When YOU
Understand
Its Language,
It May Save
Your Life!

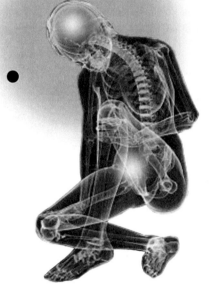

Natalie K.Y. Davis, CMT., DC Ed.

Foreword by Russell Kolbo, DC., ND.,
Certified I-ACT Colon Hydrotherapy Instructor, NBCHT Certified, Certified Wholistic Rejuvenist

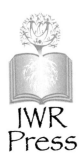

IWR
Press

Client Testimonials

"I am an elderly woman in good health and attitude. Natalie Davis has been my therapist for lymph massage and colonics for over twenty years. Visits to Natalie and the services she's provided create a result of wellness that includes a spirit of love, patience and kindness."

~ Love to You Natalie, **A. Kenney** (female)

"My experience with colon hydrotherapy occurred in the mid 90s. Due to stress from my business, my body systems were overloaded. After 2 colon hydrotherapy treatments with Natalie Davis I was amazed at the relief from the headaches and pains I experienced. Natalie is a very caring person and I am in better health due to her care."

~ **T. Myers,** (male)

"I suffered from constipation since birth. When I was in my early 30s I had a lump inside my abdomen and did not know what it was. After I studied anatomy I realized it was in the colon area. Immediately I found Natalie Davis via the Internet and scheduled for colon hydrotherapy! She coached me about how to eat and hydrate myself properly. After the therapy I felt light and I wanted to laugh all the time and, most important, the lump was gone! My abdomen looked completely different and my belly was flat for the first time in my life and my constipation was gone as well!"

~ **K. Breceljnik** (female)

BODY TALK
NEVER
LIES...

"I have been going regularly for colonics since January 1998 and have used Natalie Davis at DNS Colon Hydrotherapy since the spring of 2001 when I moved to Orange County, California. I live a healthy lifestyle, and receive many compliments about how I look much younger than my chronological age – many people guess I'm at least 10 yrs younger. I attribute this wellness to a healthy lifestyle and, specifically, taking care of myself from the inside out with colonic irrigation. Natalie is a true pro and a wealth of health information. If you want to boost your immune system and catapult your level of health to the highest, I highly recommend colonic irrigation at DNS."

~ **P. Hebda** (male)

"Natalie, I wanted to drop you a line to express how grateful I am to have found DNS Colon Hydrotherapy – your services have truly changed my life. The last 6 months have been a challenge for me, however, with your guidance, my digestive system now functions the best it ever has, and I feel terrific. Thank you for your fantastic service."

~ **C. Kimball** (female)

"Healthy regeneration is the best way to succeed. I happily and fully support Natalie Davis and her work regarding lymphatic drainage and colon hydrotherapy, which I have personally experienced many times. I work in the field of radiology and have diagnosed countless cases of varying types of cancer and disease and I don't want to 'go there'. Many health issues can be prevented, delayed and stopped by frequent internal cleansing."

~ **C.L. Holmes, M.D.** (female)

NOTE: For an in-depth case history of a very rare disease, Erythromelalgia, in the client's own words and the testimonial that follows, please refer to page 92 of this book.

Client
Testimonials

Natalie K.Y. Davis, CMT., DC Ed.
Body Talk NEVER Lies...
Copyright 1st Edition, 2012

ISBN: 978-09826524-8-0

Printed in the United States of America
Published by IWR Press
P.O. Box 1565
Sandpoint, ID 83864, USA
Publishers Email: books@iwrpress.com
Book Orders: (714) 843-2642
Author's website: www.dnscolontherapy.com
Author's Email: bodytalk@dnscolontherapy.com

Concept & Project Coordination: Dr. Gloria Gilbère
Cover and Book design: Kimberly Miller
DPI Print, Gig Harbor, WA 98335
Editing: Linda Dallmann

Publisher's Cataloguing-in-Publication Data

Davis, Natalie K. Y.
Body talk never lies ... when you understand its language, it may save your life! / Natalie K. Y. Davis, CMT., DC Ed.
     p. cm.
ISBN: 978-09826524-8-0
1. Bodywork—Transformational. 2. Colon hydrotherapy—
2. Treatment. Alternative medicine—Popular works.
I. Davis, Natalie K. Y. II. Title.
RM721 .D38 2012
615.822—dc22
     2011945831

BODY TALK
NEVER
LIES...

Contents

Foreword…

This is a book shouting to be written!

Because Natalie Davis listened to the "shouting" of her subconscious coupled with her energy and passion to share the benefits of colon hydrotherapy, her first book is now a reality.

Body Talk Never Lies will, no doubt, stimulate you to more seriously consider your own health in relation to your large intestine (colon) and the mind-body connection. This piece of literary work is of interest to lay and professional readers alike.

Colon hydrotherapy is an ancient modality (colon lavage was first recorded 3,500 years ago). Now with modern, hygienic professional devices and fully disposable colonic speculums and hosing, coupled with well-trained, competent, certified professional physicians and therapists, colon hydrotherapy is finally gaining the recognition it well deserves as a health-giving modality of therapy.

In many European countries, the field of Complimentary and Alternative Medicine (CAM) is well established, as is colon hydrotherapy, which is validated and practiced. In China and Russia, for example, it is part of the total health care system known as Integrative or Functional Medicine – as it should be in the West.

Several CAM modalities were ridiculed by the conventional western medical fraternity not long ago; now they are breaking through that glass ceiling of allopathic medicine gaining more acceptances as the benefits are becoming more and more undeniable.

I have been a naturopathic physician, chiropractor and colon hydrotherapist for more than forty years and an instructor of colon hydrotherapy for sixteen years. Tremendous progress is being made in the acceptance and teaching of colon hydrotherapy. I was instrumental in the first school for naturopathic physicians offering the course and teach it on campus along with my wife, who is also a certified instructor. I believe the only way this incredible therapy will gain the recognition it deserves is by educating more and more of our doctors who are practicing CAM principles, or are at least open to them as is the rest of the world.

Body Talk Never Lies was introduced to me by a colleague, Dr. Gloria Gilbère, a friend and author of eleven books who credits colon hydrotherapy for saving her life. She mentioned the book after the author asked her to read the manuscript for her feedback. I immediately recognized Natalie's subject matter as a potential godsend to my patients and colleagues. Its value lay in providing a potent insight for those patients who commonly manage their gastrointestinal problems through strictly dietary measures without recognizing the whole mind-body connection. They implement the high-fiber diet; the low-fat diet; the low-residue diet; the anti-yeast diet; the gluten-free diet; and other elimination diets, including the use of laxatives in order to seek some emotional and physical relief.

Based on my experience with thousands of patients, the "holistic healing" connection between the intestinal tract, known as the second brain, and the emotional brain, cannot be denied – as eloquently validated in the best-selling book *The Second Brain* by Michael E. Gerson, M.D. Up until Dr. Gerson provided scientific proof that our body actually contains a second "operating system" in our gut, phrases like "gut feelings" had no credibility – now they do, as do the case histories presented by *Body Talk Never Lies.*

Sit back, get comfortable with your favorite healthy drink and get ready for a read of a lifetime. *Body Talk Never Lies* will leave an indelible mark in how you see the mind-body connection.

– Russell Kolbo, DC, ND,
Certified I-ACT and NBCHT Colon Hydrotherapy Instructor,
Certified Wholistic Rejuvenist (CWR)

BODY TALK
NEVER
LIES...

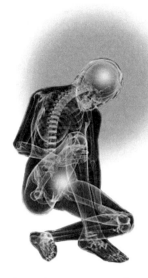

A Psychologist Speaks Out...

Bodywork is an integral part of psychotherapy. Many authors and practitioners in the field of psychology have noted the importance of observing and working with body symptoms as crucial indicators of the mind-body connection. As a psychologist of 25 years, my work has been greatly enhanced by incorporating detailed attention to my clients' complaints and concerns around their bodies. On several occasions, I have worked in teams with talented massage therapists with amazing and gratifying results.

It is for this reason I am delighted Natalie Davis has come forward with her valuable case history stories – further demonstrating the strong connection between our professional fields. Her humanistic perspective and caring attitude is reflected in the case stories that follow. They confirm the tie between Humanistic and Transformational Psychology and comparable orientations in bodywork.

The cases she presents are touching and educational. They are bound to inspire beginning and experienced therapists alike. I commend them to you for reading and to celebrate Natalie's "tender touch."

Nan White, PhD.

About the Author

Natalie K.Y. Davis, CMT., DC Ed.,

Natalie earned a doctorate in counseling education, is a certified holistic counselor, an I-ACT Certified Advanced Colon Hydrotherapy Instructor, member of I-ACT for 17 years, and a Nationally Board-certified Colon Hydrotherapist – she's been in private practice in Huntington Beach, Southern California for more than 24 years.

After performing more than 60,000 therapies she undeniably understands and validates the mind-body connection – her patient case histories don't lie anymore than the body does! The deep dark secrets uncovered by this life-enhancing therapy are sure to leave an embossed memory on those who read it – does one of her case reports resonate with situations in your life and/or practice?

Education...

- Graduate – University of Chaminade, Honolulu, Hawaii (1970)
- Graduate – University of Michigan Real Estate Program (1973)
- Post graduate – Eastern Michigan University, Industrial Tech.
- Emperor's College of Oriental Medicine, 3 years (1993)
- Graduate – Institute for Transformational Studies, Doctorate in Counseling & Education (1997)
- Colon Hydrotherapist – 24 yrs. as founder/owner/therapist of DNS MASSAGE and COLON HYDROTHERAPY (Est. 1987 to Present).
- Three-year training Program – Leola Griffin, D.C. (1987 – 2000)

BODY TALK
NEVER
LIES...

- Certificate of Completion – California Institute of Colon Hydrotherapy (1989)

Professional Affiliations/Experience...

- Member – Int'l Association for Colon Hydrotherapy (I-ACT) since 2002. Completed all levels, and earned an Advanced Instructor Certification
- Member – National Board for Colon Hydrotherapy (NBCHT) since 2009
- Holistic Health Practitioner – In Private Practice, Huntington Beach, CA, the past 24 yrs.
- Graduate – American Institute of Massage Therapy (1987)
- Certified – Sports Massage Therapy, Lymphatic Drainage Massage Therapy, Transformational Bodywork, Therapeutic Massage Therapy
- Member – American Massage Therapy Association since 1987
- State Certified – California Massage Council since 2009
- Member – National Certification Board for Therapeutic Massage and Bodywork since 1992
- Member – American Society of Alternative Therapists
- Certified – Holistic Health Counselor
- Member – Holistic Health Association since 1997

Author Contact Information...
18672 Florida St., Suite 102-A
Huntington Beach, CA 92648 USA
Clinic: (714) 843-2642
Website: www.dnscolontherapy.com

BODY TALK
NEVER
LIES...

Dedication

This book is dedicated to all Colon Hydrotherapists and the varied natural healing modalities implemented by Body Workers of the Healing Arts. Your commitment to the Transformative value of your work is forever engraved in the mind-body and soul of those you serve.

~ Thank You

BODY TALK
NEVER
LIES...

Introduction

The model of Traditional Western Medicine has always been viewed as a separation of the physical body from the mind – the non-physical mind with the belief and premise they exist independently of each other. Through time, this perception is changing as Western Medicine is coming to greater acceptance and integration of the mind-body alternative and complimentary therapies.

The Wholistic Mind-Body Approach infers there is a connection between the Mind and the Bodywork – synergistically working in concert to determine one's present state of health and well being. In turn, all thoughts and emotions affect your physical state of health and the degree of wellness and, therefore, one's mental outlook on life. This truism resonates – when we change the physiology, we also change the mentality!

Encouraging a more pro-active approach to self-care relaxation techniques and reducing stress through a plethora of bodywork modalities that include, but are not limited to, Transformational Bodywork, Therapeutic Massage, Colon Hydrotherapy, Meditation, Yoga, Exercise and Dietary changes, etc. – all contributing to greater awareness by facilitating the lowering of blood pressure, pain management, obesity, and a variety of digestive disorders such as irritable bowel syndromes.

This book addresses the question "When your body talks are you listening?" Hopefully you are, as it never lies! According to Beney Goodman, M.D., "With the attention to the body at an all time high, we are increasingly likely to express emotional discomfort in a physical rather than a verbal language." (Jan/Feb 1995 Psychology Today, pg.26)

The writing of this book is also expressly poised to achieve the following:

- To relate authentic stories of client experiences through the body modalities of Colon Hydrotherapy, Therapeutic Massage and Transformational Bodywork.

- To help readers mirror their own emotional and physical experiences through these case histories and the related bodywork modalities employed that brought about the change or realization of some underlying causes.

- To express and explore the extraordinary combination of these modalities and their therapeutic benefits: cleansing, detoxifying and dispelling old emotional holding patterns through facilitating bowel elimination.

I have always believed that the way we eat and eliminate is a microcosm of the way we live our lives – if we are eating and eliminating well, we are moving with the flow of life!

If however, we are constipated, consider that we are stuck in the past and thus old holding patterns are formed, inhibiting our ability to eliminate. Impacted bowels are a metaphor for holding onto past traumas and subconscious stories that continue to have an emotional charge!

The inability to let go of the past, especially unresolved issues, causes suppressed anger, fear and sadness that often lead to anxiety and depression.

Many of us learned early on that when life gets chaotic and untrusting, the only way to have some semblance of control was to control our bowels. We can decide to eliminate or not, and these early patterns extend into adulthood.

The voluntary nervous system affects our digestive tract – from our mouth to our anus. When our body talks to us, it talks by way of sounds, flatulence and gurgling noises. The body lets us know when we are hungry or satiated. The forming of gas and bloating are part of the vocabulary of our body. It knows if we ate badly by "speaking" to us like if there is an intestinal backup with an accompanying dull ache – it's trying to get your attention!

BODY TALK
NEVER
LIES...

I remember one particular client who comes to mind, who experienced bowel sounds like "an old creaky door that opened in a mystery movie!" – prompting her to have colon hydrotherapy.

Our body talks to us physically by way of symptoms – pain is a manifestation the body is seeking our attention. The pain will increase with intensity until it gets our fullest attention until it gets so unbearable we must seek help! The mind can only ignore it for so long and the body pain usually prevails, until we look at the root cause underlying our symptoms. The pain is the signal calling to action – when your body talks it never lies!

When we are nervous or upset, the body will often manifest a facial tick or the twitching of a leg noting our impatience. It is also common to hear someone say, "My stomach is in knots!" – an expression of our fear or nervous energy. The mind and body is in constant communication – when our body talks, we need to learn to listen!

As a body worker and colon hydrotherapist of 24 years, learning to read the body has become second nature to me. It is with clear intention, that I begin each and every session with the awareness that I am only the facilitator – directed by a Divine Spirit intuitively moving within a process of deep awakening through the client's ability to become authentic with his or her self.

As a therapist, you nurture a great deal of compassion for yourself and others in doing bodywork in any modality. When connecting with your clients, do so in such a way that you're absolutely devoid of any judgment. When a therapist allows their own "stuff" to get in the way, judgment will separate you from those you can potentially help! When you come from your heart, openness and acceptance will allow you to see their true essence. Then and only then, you can be the catalyst for their transformation and change.

BODY TALK
NEVER
LIES...

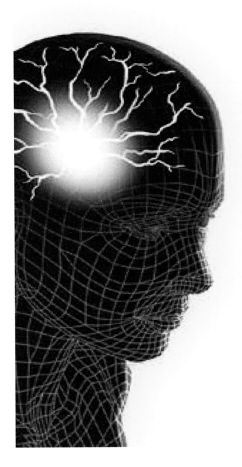

Finding Life's Purpose

When I was ten years old, I attended a Saturday afternoon matinee at the Princess Theater with my brother Doug. From the corner of my eye, I noticed a stranger sitting six seats away to my right. I was absorbed in the movie "Ben Hur" with Charlton Heston playing the lead role. Oddly, I had noticed the man getting closer and closer to me, until he was sitting right next to me. Suddenly, he started groping my right thigh. I quickly stood up and shouted to my brother to move down to another seat because this man was grabbing my leg and thigh. The molester immediately left the theater and without thinking too much about the incident, I went back to watching the movie.

At age 40 (thirty years later), while receiving a therapeutic massage, the therapist was working on my right thigh and I experienced a memory flash back to my encounter at the movie theater. This was the first time I realized, through cellular memory, that the mind and body connection was very real! This clarity subsequently led me to Transformational Bodywork and to helping others discover what cellular memories may have shaped their lives and, possibly, inhibited their truth in becoming authentic with their self.

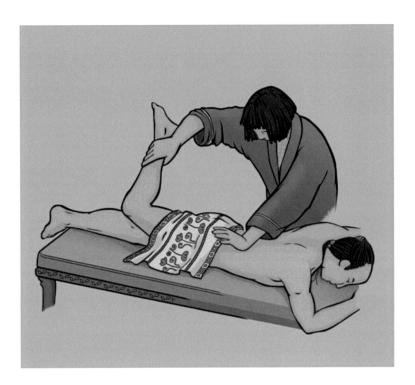

Tuina

In spring of 1988, I had the opportunity to be one of sixteen massage therapists from the U.S. to go to Beijing, China and study at the National Institute of Sports Science. This was part of a student exchange program, where we worked on China's Olympic Athletes and learned a methodology called "Tuina" – the name for the "pushing and pulling" massage technique used in China effectively for thousands of years. Even today in many Chinese hospitals a floor is dedicated to this modality and, in most cases, used as a precursor before any surgery. Surgery being the very last resort!

The Beijing program lasted for six weeks. On alternating days, we went from the inpatient hospital to train and the following day the outpatient clinic.

While sitting in the bus one day, a woman in her thirties, from Zurich, Switzerland joined our group. She was a physical therapist and thought the Tuina Program would enhance her work. She chose to sit next to me and before too long she nudged me and asked me, "Can you help me?"

I responded, "What's wrong?"

The woman said, "I cannot go!"

Quizzically, I responded, "Meaning you cannot move your bowels or eliminate?"

She nodded yes; I then asked her how many days she had been in this distress without being able to evacuate her bowels. She proceeded to show me 7 fingers, meaning 7 days. "Is there something you can do to help me?"

I replied, "Yes, there is something I can do, but you'll need to wait until we return to the hotel!"

Upon returning, I went back to my hotel room and retrieved my aromatherapy oils, that I had packed for this trip but couldn't help but wonder how this woman could possibly know to sit next to me, not knowing that I was also a colon hydrotherapist as well as a massage therapist. I've since come to the conclusion that we are divinely led at all times.

I went to the woman's room and immediately poured two glasses of hot water out of the thermos to cool. The tap water in China had too many microbes making it impossible to drink out of the faucet. The hotel staff would bring us boiling hot water to fill the thermos in the room every morning.

I proceeded to employ some of my manual colon massage and Tuina techniques I had learned. After the first 15 minutes, I gave her the first glass of water to drink followed by another and then replenished the glasses with more hot water to cool so she could drink. I continued to massage her abdomen for a total of 45 minutes, with the instruction to finish the 7th and 8th glass of water. In that short time, her abdomen transformed from the hardness of a basketball, to being softer and supple. I told her, she would be evacuating her bowels within an hour!

The following morning, while waiting in the bus to leave for the outpatient clinic, the woman comes running to the bus calling out my name, "Natalie, Natalie you've saved my life!"

I asked her, "How do you feel?"

She replied, "Oh let me tell you, it was like a volcano eruption! How did you know that I would eliminate within an hour?"

It was that sudden moment, with amazing clarity, that I realized I could go anywhere in the world and make a living with my hands. But more importantly, I was following my life's purpose and my gifted spiritual path that combines the healing modalities of massage and colon hydrotherapy.

I then reflected on my childhood memory of being one of 9 children. Once a month my mother lined all of us up in a row and force-fed each of us a big tablespoon of Phillip's Milk of Magnesia©! This was my earliest experience with intestinal cleansing – my mother's way of reducing illness in a large family. Look at me now, I've professionalized it and, thank God, she is still alive to have witnessed it.

Tuina

23

BODY TALK
NEVER
LIES...

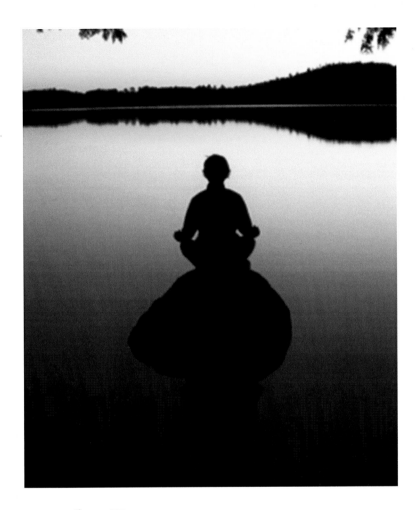

Body Reverence

Each morning upon rising I thank God for another day and welcome the newness of what the day will bring! I also thank God for the love of family and friends in my life and for passion in the bodywork that has served me well for 24 years. There is a joy with humility each time I go to my office knowing I'm just the facilitator and that God is working through me – creating a safe place for everyone to unload their burdens and feel relaxation and renewal.

Reverence is defined as: a feeling of profound awe or attitude of deep respect and often love for something sacred. As a body worker, having reverence for the body is so important because it sets the tone of the work that follows. In touching someone, you are also touched back – an energetic exchange and sacredness in honoring the person laying on the massage table as the bodywork begins. The example of reverence for the body is displayed in the form of the Hawaiian Culture's Huna Healing – a process of bodywork that is continuous for 3 days, as boy becomes a man, an initiation and sacred rites of passage!

BODY TALK
NEVER
LIES...

26

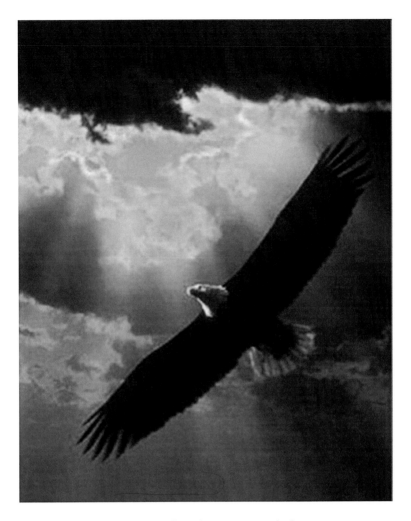

Journey of the Self

Transformational Bodywork training was a rite-of-passage for me with Fred and Cheryl Mitouer, owners and educators of the Pacific School of Healing Arts in Gualala, California since 1988.   I went from a conventional medical massage background to incorporating an eclectic spiritual massage. This integration of both modalities heightened my awareness and I came to trust the transformative value of the process in doing the work, which has shaped who I am today.

Transformational Bodywork is as much a professional training program consisting of seven levels of in depth healing aspects as well as an art form of personal disarmament. This is a process that strips away the holding patterns within the body musculature and taps into the unhealed wounds of cellular memory, which continue to hold onto an emotional charge. This training attracts the gifted and mature practitioners of the healing arts. Psychotherapy, spiritual disciplines, and body workers whose work will be greatly enhanced by living more consciously – it is the Soul's journey of discovering the Essence of the authentic self for both the client and therapist.

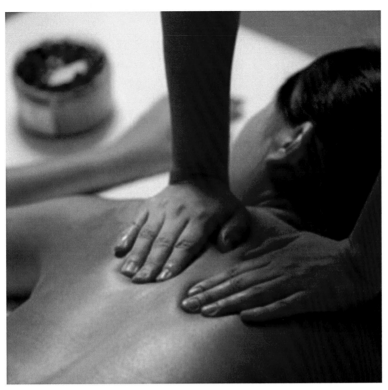

What is Transformational Bodywork?

A Transformational Bodywork session is unlike any other form of healing modality – it is usually 2 hours long and often longer. Atypical in that one does not start out seeking relaxation and calmness, yet it becomes a consequence of the end result of the session – becoming a process of self discovery and a deep exploration and purging from the psyche and musculature holding patterns that continue to run, thus shaping our behavior. It is the process of revealing unhealed wounds and traumas that hold an emotional charge through cellular memory. The experienced therapist is able to read these holding patterns in the body's armor and through various deep tissue techniques – bringing about a softening to those hardened contracted muscle layers.

Transformational Bodywork integrates both breath work and acupressure to open up the meridians of the body and get the energetic flow moving past any blockages.

After the Transformational Bodywork session, the client is able to feel every pulsation riveting throughout his or her body. There is aliveness the client has, more than likely, never before felt! It feels like you have had the best cry of your life with complete surrender and insight to your suffering with amazing clarity!

Personally, my experience with Transformational Bodywork has been profoundly life changing! It has heightened my awareness to live more consciously, authentically and in the moment!

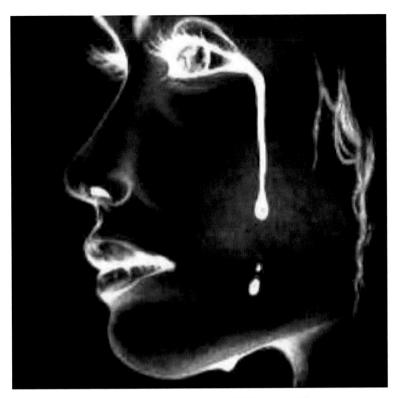

Speaking Your Truth

The following is a case history of Transformational Bodywork that may resonate to most of us who have been in relationships or marriages that were abusive (mentally and/or physically) and controlling.

A 43 year old woman was referred to me for Transformational Bodywork. Her stature was 5'1" and all of 105 pounds. She appeared to be very mild mannered, but repressed her anger towards a controlling husband of 18 years. She was not able to speak her truth and stand up for herself. It was a frightening task to confront her husband when he was angry. He was 6'4" and weighed 450 pounds, which alone was intimidating.

As the work proceeded, my assessments of the client's areas of holding patterns were in her neck, jaw and back. The area of the neck was very contracted with the neck rotators being extremely tight – limiting her range of motion in turning side to side. Metaphysically, it also represented the lack of extension and the inability to take risks – like a turtle that recoils its neck to protect itself when it feels threatened and extends its neck when it feels safe. Her chronic low back pain indicated the lack of support. The jaw area was also interestingly in a tight holding pattern – limiting her ability to project the sound of her voice and speak what she really felt and also indicated the stuffing of one's pride! I worked to lengthen the inner pterygoid muscles of her mouth with the caution that I would not take any responsibility for whatever she would say. The client derived so many insights from her cathartic session she commented upon leaving my office that she felt lighter and self-empowered and in touch with a new sense of autonomous freedom she had not felt before!

The following morning I received a phone call from her husband, in his loud inquiring voice saying, "What did you do to my wife? In 18 years of marriage she has never raised her voice to me and now she told me off in many ways – it's like you have unleashed a dragon that I never knew was there! Whatever you did to my wife, I want the same kind of bodywork and need to make an appointment with you."

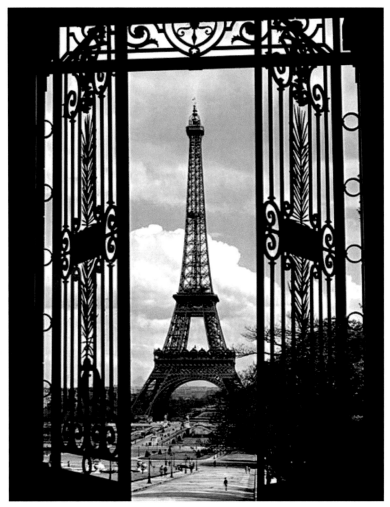

A "Towering" Validation

In January 1993, I received a phone call from Paris, France from a client who previously lived in San Diego, California, and saw me for Transformational Bodywork. She was now living in Paris and asked, "Natalie how many people would it take for you to fly to Paris to do some Transformational Bodywork; there is no one doing it here?"

My response was, "Are you serious?"

"Yes, I am!" she replied.

I meditated on her inquiry and replied, "I'll need 20 people for 2-hour sessions each."

She said, "Just let me know the time and date of your arrival; I'll arrange it!"

The days and weeks passed, the time neared to my travel to Paris and everything fell into place. My schedule was arranged to allow me to go. In addition, United Airlines had its first round-trip available for first class, non-stop from Los Angeles to Paris for a mere $400 – the synchronicity of events validated to me that I was definitely meant to go and I departed in March of that year!

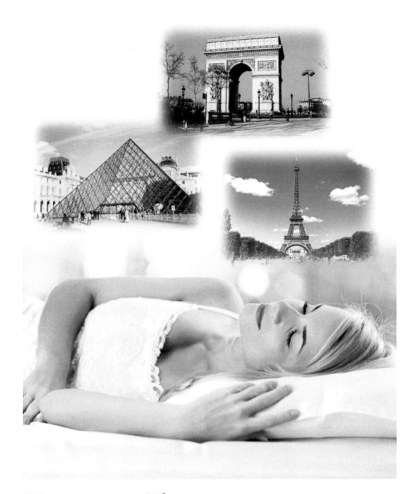

Dream Chatter

I had a series of recurring dreams prior to my departure to Paris. I dreamt six times in living color and it would always start and end the same. The dream began with seeing myself being picked up at the Charles De Gaulle Airport by a tiny white car – my suitcase was so big that it stuck out the back window. As the car made its way through the streets of Paris, we passed the Arc de Triomphe onto the stone cobbled streets in the 5th Arondismont (district).

As the dream continued, I saw a very old historical-type four-story stone block building with a black mansard roof and black ornate wrought iron balconies with French doors housing glass panes that opened from ceiling to floor. I saw myself get out of the car and walk up to a set of green doors then up many steps.

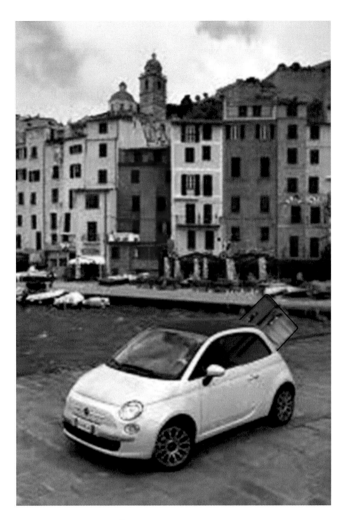

Arrival in Paris

Finally, the auspicious day of arrival in Paris was at hand. I was met by my client at the airport, and, to my amazement, she drove a tiny white Fiat, which I had no way of knowing she had, as it was never mentioned. The Fiat barely fit two people, let alone my suitcase. It was so large it had to stick out the back window.

As she continued to drive through the streets of Paris, we passed the Arc de Triomphe and I was thinking, "God, it's like I'm living my dream!" The car finally came to a stop in front of a building, which exactly fit the description of what I witnessed in my dream. I asked my client, "How old would you say these buildings are?"

She replied, "Well, they had to have been built back around the early 1800s." – this WAS definitely déjà vu!
I had subconsciously transported myself from my dream state to actually see a preview of what was to come!

I got out of the car, now anticipating the forest green colored front doors as I had seen in my dream. I proceeded to walk up the wide oak steps worn by time and the thousands of shoe impressions over many centuries that preceded me. There were no elevators! There were two dimly lit sconces along the wall, with just enough light to help prevent tripping while ascending the steps to apartment #13.

BODY TALK
NEVER
LIES...

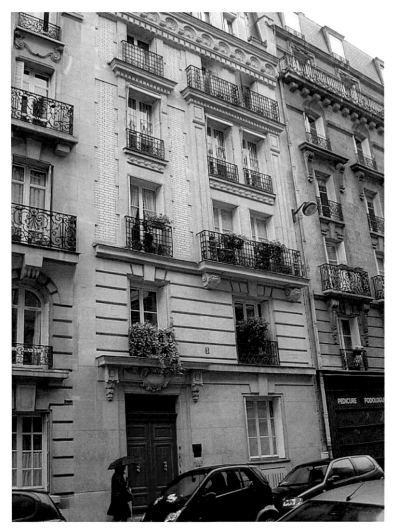

The Journey Continues...

Over the course of my two weeks in Paris, I worked and stayed in this small studio apartment that was provided me by my host. The bathroom was at the very top of the third level of steps, and the attic space contained a makeshift shower. It took climbing another set of steps to reach the lofted area, where I slept on a futon. There was a tiny kitchen no more than four feet wide reeking strongly of the garlic sitting on the counter.

Over the coming days, I was to experience things that my massage and bodywork career could have never imagined! That said, I trusted my abilities and approached my work at hand with no fear or apprehension – I knew I could handle whatever showed up!

I was told there was an entire subculture of a million U.S. expatriates living in Paris and they were yearning for Transformational Bodywork.

BODY TALK
NEVER
LIES...

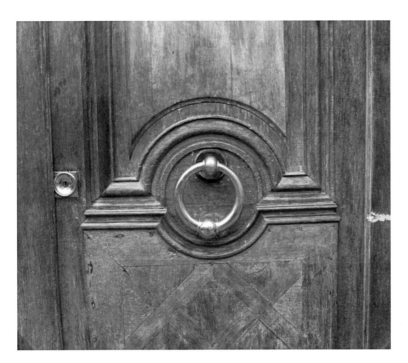

First Encounter

A forty year old woman presented at my door at her appointed time. I asked her, "What are your particular issues?" to which she replied, "I have these smells...I can't quite describe them to you!"

I inquired, "When do these smells present themselves?"

She replied, "They come any time of the day! It doesn't matter what I'm doing, I can be lying in bed reading a book, or I can be working on a client and this wafting smell comes over me!"

"Can you tell me what it smells like?"

She hesitated a moment and then replied, "It smells like rotting flesh!"

As she lay on the massage table, I approached her body with reverence and humility and began with a silent prayer asking the Holy Spirit to guide me through this woman's processes. My intentions were clear and pure of heart – simply to facilitate her transformation. I had asked her to do some continuous deep breathing while I opened the meridians of her body through a series of acupressure points. After some time passed, she curled up in a fetal position and began making animal like sounds – snorting pig-like sounds! There was a curious aura of what appeared to be like horns projecting from the top of her head... and her tongue had literally turned purple in color. At this time, I felt the presence of a spirit or an entity within her... followed by a cold shiver up my spine. Intuitively, I shouted, "Be gone!" Suddenly the two windows that were

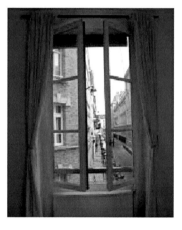

slightly parted completely blew wide open simultaneously from inside-out as if there was a sudden gust of wind within the room pushing both windows out. I kept a firm presence and focus and continued the bodywork. After two hours of applying energetic therapy, I was spent!

At the end of our session, she commented that she felt lighter; she thanked me and proceeded on her way. Three weeks after returning to the U.S. I received a letter from this woman. She thanked me for the incredible work. She said I had transformed her and she no longer smelled those strong smells... and the entities she felt had left! This bordered on the bizarre, and was the first in my career, as I had never experienced anything that could be categorized as an actual exorcism!

I felt the power of God protected me. I also believe that the pungent smell of garlic that permeated the room shielded me from something even more sinister.

BODY TALK
NEVER
LIES...

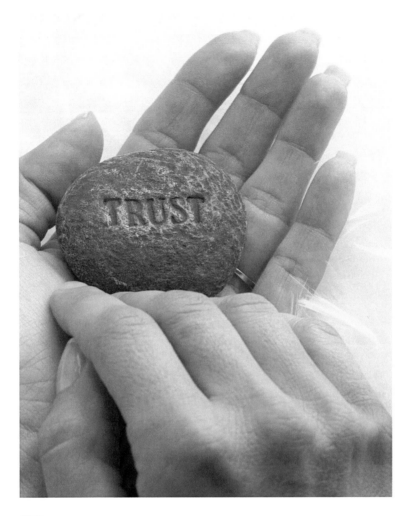

Trust

Trust is essential to the process of any bodywork modality – the client and therapist relationship MUST be based on complete trust, tantamount to a good outcome in every session. When a new client arrives and is greeted a rapport is established within the first ten minutes, no matter what the services are that are being offered.

Massage and colon hydrotherapy are becoming more accepted mainstream modalities. By taking the time to educate the client about the process before one begins, knowledge will relieve any fears and apprehensions. If the client is referred by someone they know and trust, they are more likely to embrace and trust the process and the therapist.

As a body worker, I have never experienced apprehension from any client that I couldn't handle! However, on several occasions, I have referred a client to another health professional when the problem/challenge was bigger than what I knew I could offer them. The following case will demonstrate this point! As a body worker, I believe it is necessary to be in alignment with the integrity of what you do! I, too, receive massages and colon hydrotherapy.

We profess health, so therefore we must have a healthy regimen ourselves! If we practice what we teach and apply, it further reinforces their trust in the therapist. Through our own cleansing and detoxification, we become clearer and set the intention for our own wellness.

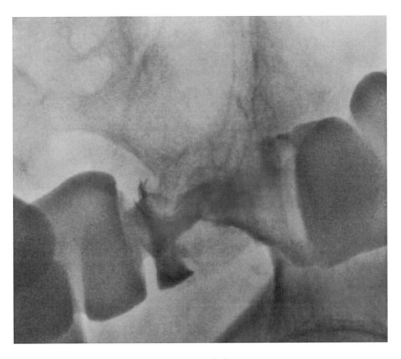

Hitting a Wall

This is a case of a fifty-four year old gentlemen, who had been coming to me for both massage and colon hydrotherapy a number of years. He sold his thriving practice as an attorney and moved to France – realizing his life-long dream of living as a Frenchman!

One year passed and he returned to California and made an appointment with me for colon hydrotherapy. During his session, I could barely administer 20 ounces of water before "hitting a wall!" After repeated fills it always ended the same – a wet pad. At that juncture, I instructed him to take 4 tablespoons of mineral oil and return the next day.

The following day, upon palpating the left descending colon, I felt a lump the size of a lemon and asked him, "Have you ever noticed this lump before?"

He replied, "Not until now that you bring it to my attention!" I continued his colon hydrotherapy and filled very slowly. I still could not get past that wall of matter. I commented that it appeared he has a holding pattern here and it might be a blockage! I proceeded to refer him to a gastroenterologist.

I asked him to be sure and share with me what the specialist found. Ten days later, he called me to say, "Do you want the bad news or good news first?"

I replied, "Give me the bad news first!"

He continued, "I went to the gastroenterologist as you advised and he did discover a lemon-size mass! The biopsy showed it was a malignant cancer! The good news is that I don't have to wear a bag! The doctor said that once they do the colon resection they can do what is known as an anastomosis, which connects the bowel to the rectum."

I asked, "When are you scheduled for surgery?"

He replied, "Next week Tuesday!"

On Thursday, after my early morning tennis game, I stopped at the hospital and visited with him; he was talkative and vibrant! I rested assured he was doing well!

I went out of town for the weekend to attend a conference. On Monday morning, upon returning to my office, a recorded message said they were having a memorial service for him. As you can imagine, I was shocked! How could this be? Apparently, after the surgery, his blood became sepsis, hit his brain and killed him.

Clearly this was a situation that was too big for me to handle, and it was important for me to refer him to someone who could help him – it's unfortunate that the diagnosis and surgery led to his demise! That said, this case history speaks loud and clear to the importance of colon hydrotherapy as a prevention of colon cancer with a timely colonoscopy by age 50 as a base-line marker.

BODY TALK
NEVER
LIES...

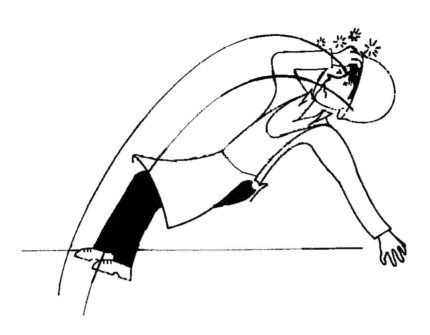

Physically Present ~ Mentally Absent

As a colon hydrotherapist, I've had my share of difficult cases, some much more than others! The next case history I share has to do with the degree of disassociation – defined as a perceived detachment of the mind from the emotional state or even the body. Some people are not in their body, they may be physically present but mentally absent – many times as a coping mechanism for some past trauma!

I recount to you the story of a forty-five year old woman who had come to me due to chronic constipation. Her bowel eliminations were so difficult that they resulted in her fainting while sitting on the commode. While unconscious, she was relaxed enough to have an involuntary evacuation of her bowel. Providing a bit of family history will lend insight to her difficult bowel pattern.

Her mother died of a brain aneurysm while sitting on the commode when this patient was a teenager. Her father also died while sitting on the toilet from a blockage to the main carotid artery. In her mind, she associated bowel elimination with dying!

I proceeded very slowly with the colon hydrotherapy – respecting there was a great deal of anxiety and fear. Repeatedly, in a calming voice, I instructed her to open her eyes and stay in the present moment – reassuring her she would get through this and everything would be all right! I continued to remind her to breathe, followed by more reassurance! The colon hydrotherapy process was a series of short water fills and releases.

The second day, I continued the disarming process keeping her eyes open and staying present of mind and in her body. The colon hydrotherapy continued slowly with again a series of short fills and releases!

By the third session she started releasing fecal matter, and up to this time she could not even look at it being expelled through the enclosed viewing tube – there was so much unconscious denial! I see that denial is true-to-form with clients who are disassociated from their bodies.

By the fourth and fifth session she was able to accept longer fills of water and released more with less fear.

I followed her progress through weekly phone calls – she was now having regular bowel movements without any reoccurrence of fainting.

BODY TALK
NEVER
LIES...

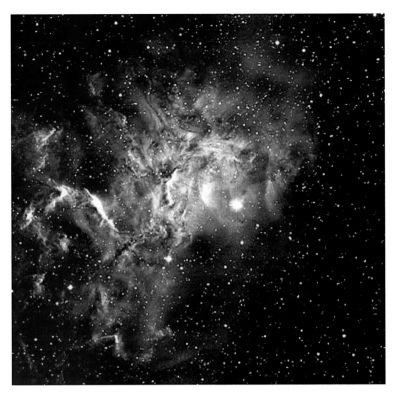

Metaphysically Speaking...

The Mind-Body-Spirit is ever so connected to our overall physical state of being. I've always believed and witnessed that the symptoms manifest in the weakest area of the body. The solar plexus, which doctors call the "celiac plexus," is a juncture point of nerves in the abdomen, near the stomach. Many medical culture's (ancient and current) believe it is the center of intuition and the seat of emotions. Conventional medical science has found that the celiac plexus is a vulnerable point, where the interconnecting nerves can be irritated, causing pain. Thus, it is also a convenient point to relieve pain.

The solar plexus is also known as our power center, and when our survival is threatened, often the "fight or flight" defense kicks in! The emotional response to this holding of anger would reflect the colon's ability/inability to eliminate. The more repressed the emotional anger the more it may lead to irritable bowel or ulcerative colitis, for example. This next case demonstrates this point, as it was necessary to go beyond the physical, the mind, and the spirit to facilitate the healing processes!

Nerves involved in the solar plexus include those that govern the autonomic nervous system – that part of the nervous system that we don't voluntarily control. The autonomic nervous system regulates organ function, constriction and dilation of blood vessels and pupil size, for example.

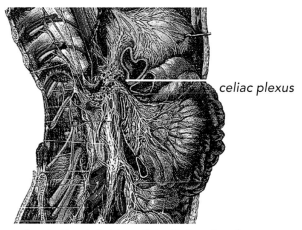

celiac plexus

According to the definition of the University of Pittsburgh, the solar plexus, or celiac plexus, is a bundle of nerves crossing in the abdomen.

Plexus simply means "network," and scores of these nerve networks twine throughout the body. If you've ever had the wind knocked out of you, that's an effect of a blow to the celiac plexus. The blow irritates a nerve in the nearby diaphragm, causing it to spasm. Since the diaphragm is essential to breathing, you can't breathe until the effect wears off.

Metaphysical is a word that, often times, is misunderstood and thereby inappropriate connotations are relayed from it. My hope, in providing the following definition, is that you will have a greater understanding of its meanings as a type of philosophy that uses broad concepts to help define reality and our understanding of it – it is not a methodology based in any religious genre.

Derived from the Greek meta ta physika ("after the things of nature") – referring to an idea, doctrine, or posited reality outside of human sense perception. In modern philosophical terminology, metaphysics refers to the studies of what cannot be reached through objective studies of material reality.

Metaphysical studies generally seek to explain inherent or universal elements of reality, which are not easily discovered or experienced in our everyday life. As such, it is concerned with explaining the features of reality that exist beyond the physical world and our immediate senses. Metaphysics, therefore, uses logic based on the meaning of human terms, rather than on a logic tied to human sense perception of the objective world. Metaphysics might include the study of the nature of the human mind, the definition and meaning of existence, or the nature of space, time, and/or causality.

The origin of philosophy, beginning with the Pre-Socratics, was metaphysical in nature. For example, the philosopher Plotinus held that the reason in the world and in the rational human mind is only a reflection of a more universal and perfect reality beyond our limited human reason. He termed this ordering power in the universe "God."

Metaphysical ideas, because they are not based on direct experience with material reality, are often in conflict with the modern sciences. Beginning with the Enlightenment and the Scientific Revolution, experiments with, and observations of, the world became the yardsticks for measuring truth and reality. Therefore, our contemporary valuation of scientific knowledge over other forms of knowledge helps explain the controversy and skepticism concerning metaphysical claims, which are considered unverifiable by modern science.

In matters of religion, the problem of validating metaphysical claims is most readily seen in all of the "proofs" for the existence of God. Like trying to prove the existence of a "soul" or "spirit" in the human, attempts to scientifically prove the existence of God and other nonobjective, nonhuman realities is seemingly impossible. The difficulty arises out of the attempt to scientifically study and objectify something, which, by its very nature, cannot become an object of our scientific studies. This reigning belief that everything can be explained scientifically in terms of natural causes - referred to as naturalism - compels many to think that only what is seen or sensed, only what can be hypothesized and tested can be true, and therefore, meaningful to us as humans.

Recently, however, even as metaphysics has come under attack for its apparent lack of access to real knowledge, so has science begun to have its own difficulties in claiming absolute knowledge. Continual developments in our understanding of the human thought process reveals that science cannot solely be relied upon to explain reality, for the human mind cannot be seen as simply a mirror of the natural world. For example, since the act of scientific observation itself tends to produce the reality it hopes to explain, the so-called "truths" of science cannot be considered as final or objective. This fact manifests itself over and over again, as scientific truths and laws continue to break down or yield to new and better explanations of reality. What becomes apparent, therefore, is that the process of human interpretation in the sciences, as elsewhere, is both variable and relative to the observer's viewpoint.

Metaphysically
Speaking...

BODY TALK
NEVER
LIES...

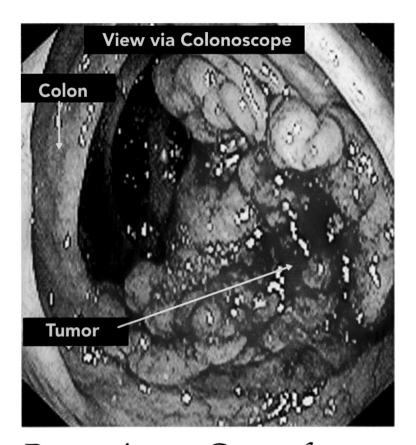

Reversing a Case of Ulcerative Colitis, Naturally

This is a story of a man in his mid-forties who was referred to me because of a chronic case of ulcerative colitis. His condition was so severe it resulted in seventeen episodes a day necessitating evacuation of his bowel accompanied with bleeding. His gastroenterologist was ready to remove his entire colon! Since we know that colon hydrotherapy is contraindicated for this condition, I focused first on his nutrition and had him eliminate the acidic foods in his diet, more particularly, the nightshades (potatoes, tomatoes, eggplant, peppers, paprika, cayenne, etc.) as they have been scientifically validated as contributing to an existing inflammatory process. He additionally reduced his intake of alcohol and caffeine and increased his water consumption. I also recommended he consume four tablespoons of flaxseed oil daily to enterically coat the walls of his colon to assist in buffering the irritation. I suggested some fiber and a high-potency probiotic supplement to begin supporting his intestinal health. When taken together, they move through the colon coating the walls and begin the colonizing of good bacteria to facilitate healing of colonic ulcerations. He continued on the recommended supplements for 45 days and during that time went from bowel eliminations of seventeen times daily to two normal daily bowel movements. Once the bleeding from his colon stopped most of his anxiety was eliminated.

I suggested to him that while I focus on the nutritive aspects of his care it is also important for him to address any repressed anger issues by seeking counsel from a psychotherapist who can help deal with the emotional component as it relates to ulcerative colitis. He confirmed to me that he was one that did not like to talk about his feelings! After that comment I replied, "Unless you deal with this issue, you will never be totally free from this debilitating condition!"

I proceeded slowly with his first session of colon hydrotherapy and provided him with plenty of reassurance. His second colon hydrotherapy was the next day – at no time did the client show any signs of internal bleeding. I was confident the fiber supplements were working because he reported his stools were well formed and bowels were

BODY TALK
NEVER
LIES...

normally moving two times per day by the sixth session of his colon hydrotherapy. He continued with a once a month maintenance session for the next seven months. I suggested he have another colonoscopy and confirm how his colon had changed!

After his colonoscopy, his gastroenterologist went over the results with him. The doctor asked, "What have you been doing? Nine months ago we were ready to remove your colon! There are now NO ulcerations on the walls of your colon... it's as if you have the colon of a twenty-five year old!"

My client shared that he had changed his diet and was having colon hydrotherapy and counseling. His doctor replied, "Whatever you're doing continue with it because your colon is completely healed!"

Once my client had confirmation from his doctor that his colon was now indeed healed, he could move forward with his life without the fear hanging over him that he might have to live without a colon! His past condition had severely inhibited his personal and professional life. To say the least, he was elated and very grateful. A few days later, I received a large gift basket of fruit and a personal note thanking me! It was so rewarding knowing this client's colon was saved and I helped facilitate the therapies that made that possible!

Reversing a Case of
Ulcerative Colitis, Naturally

BODY TALK
NEVER
LIES...

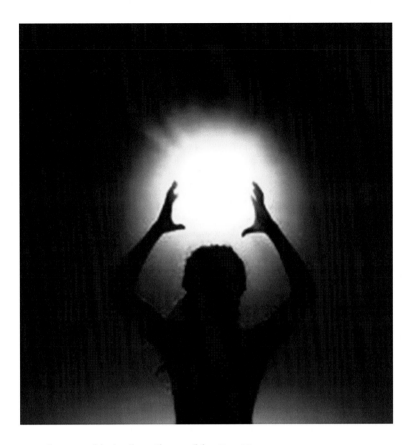

The "Ah ha" Moment

This next story is evidence of how the mind-body-connection is so powerful! I believe, in performing any body modality – massage or colon hydrotherapy – one can access the underlying emotion that is "stuck" in a holding pattern.

It is imperative to ask the clients' permission before going down the bodywork path – they may feel vulnerable and be more resistant to sharing their emotions as they reveal aspects of their personal lives. Holding patterns in the colon are formed as a need to stay in control, including cases of chronic constipation!

A 42 year old woman suffering from chronic constipation came to me for colon hydrotherapy. After 20 minutes into the session she was still not releasing and was in a definite holding pattern. So I asked her for permission to explore and look at, "What's going on? You're in a holding pattern in your colon and experience tells me there's a specific emotion behind it?"

She replied, "Yes, I would like to know!"

So I instructed her to close her eyes – this type of bodywork often moves intuitively! I placed my hand on her abdomen, more particularly the area of her descending colon, and said to her, "Bring your focus here and specifically to the word 'nurturing'." Then I asked, "What do you consider the most nurturing aspect of your life?"

What seemed like 3 minutes of silence went by as she started welling up with tears and her face became flushed as she held back a flood of emotions! I then gave her permission to cry, "You know release takes many forms, including crying! Where is this emotion coming from, what is the picture behind the emotion?"

By this time the tears were flowing and her crying lasted several minutes. During this time, the colonic waste hose and viewing tube was full! She continued a deep and agonizing cry while simultaneously releasing more and more fecal matter!

"What is the subconscious picture?" I asked.

She finally replied, "I'm about three years of age and I'm in a crib-like bed. I have pooped in my pants and I am now spreading it on the walls!"

I asked, "Where is your mother in all this?"

She said, "She's standing by the door!" I then instructed her to zoom into her memory like a camera lens with her mind's eye and especially pay attention to her mother's facial expression.

She continued to emote with more tears, "My mother is very loving and nurturing!"

There we go, the buzzword that made the connection to the holding pattern and cellular memory of the past!

"She's coming in with a towel to clean me up!" More tears were shed as she continued to release with so much peristalsis that her evacuation is flowing out of the tube.

I said, "Now I want you to draw inward and see the insight for what it is – bring in your psychology experience now and recognize that the association of your mother's love and nurturance is being revisited every time there is constipation!"

Still tearing she said, "This was the last vision of my mother because she died in an automobile crash and I was raised by nannies and my father so I never did know my mother very well!"

Now it became evident to us both that she had held on to the last memory of her mother – her mother's love and nurturing!

At the end of our session, she gave me a big hug and told me, "You don't know how much you have helped me Natalie! I've been in psychoanalysis twelve years and no one has ever touched upon this aspect!"

I replied, "I'm just your facilitator; you were now ready to let this go!" This was her awakening process.

As colon hydrotherapists and body workers, we know that as we create a safe place, the client's "body armor" will breakdown and release the underlying emotional issue, which has been buried for years. This "ah ha" moment of discovery becomes pivotal to change the old holding patterns and bio-defense mechanisms. The transformative value of the work becomes so profound and intimately tied to accessing emotionally charged unconscious patterns within the physical body. In this case, she was freed her of chronic constipation!

The "Ah ha"
Moment

BODY TALK
NEVER
LIES...

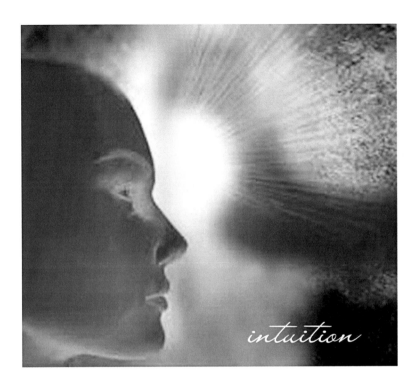

intuition

"Gut" Intuition

Intuition is that inspired knowing that often is coined as a 6th sense – a gut-level feeling fueled by our inner knowledge that goes beyond hunches. It is being able to sense truth from a gut instinct and listening from a place of inner vision and dialog. It's allowing the mystery of life to unfold, rather than trying to make things happen with specific expectations!

Intuition is a heartfelt guidance that gets sharper and more exacting the more we use it. I believe everyone has an intuitive ability – some more than most will tap into it by way of gut feelings and emotions.

As a body worker, through the intuitive sense of touch

coupled with a working knowledge of the body, one is able to read and access the holding patterns within the physical body that affects unconscious beliefs that hold an emotional charge. This is a subtle form of body talk as the body holds cellular memories and biological defense mechanisms are manifested in the musculature.

This next case history is about a 42 year old woman who came to see me for massage therapy. After working with her for the second time, I asked her throughout the session to take several deep breaths. There was a noticeable rattle-like sound in her inhalation that I detected and it did not sound right to me! This was her body's way of talking and telling me there was a problem – I listened! I was compelled to tell her that something was not quite right with her respiration. During the massage I asked her if she had a complete physical exam recently. She told me she had had a physical within the last six months, and that she checked out fine – everything was within "normal" range. To which I responded, "That was then and this is now, and I am really compelled to tell you that you need to see your doctor to have this rattle sound checked out! I believe you have a problem affecting your respiration! Please do not wait! Call me and let me know what they find?"

Ten days later, I received a phone call from the client. She said, "You know Natalie you're the first person to have said anything or pinpoint some physical problem with me. After many years of physical exams there have been no problems found until now!" After her physical exam, they did some further testing and found a fifty-cent size hole in her heart – causing her to generate four times the amount of oxygenated blood. That condition was affecting her respiration and responsible for the rattle sound I detected.

She commented, "I was a walking time bomb, ready to explode; you saved my life."

BODY TALK
NEVER
LIES...

The correct diagnosis was achieved simply by advising her to seek a medical exam and to have further testing. She was scheduled for open-heart surgery the following week!

After eight weeks, I followed up with a visit to her home and brought in some of her favorite Chinese food. While sitting on her couch having lunch, she commented, "You know, I can't figure out why there is a bruise under my left foot?"

"Let me see." I looked under her foot; the bruise was at the heart reflex point of the foot. Now the bruise made complete sense because she had just had open-heart surgery and there is considerable bruising of the heart in repairing the hole.

The human body is so amazing! The bruise on her left foot connected to the heart organ of her body, reconfirming the validity of reflexology as a science, as the Chinese have known and practiced for centuries. The body talks to us, when it does we need to listen – it never lies! As body workers and therapists, we build a close relationship to people through touch. In doing so, we cannot help but be touched back – there IS an energetic exchange that is undeniable! I often find myself so attune with my clients that after a number of sessions – weekly, monthly or semi-monthly, I am able to pick up on the subtlest changes in that particular client's body or energy.

As body workers, we are the first responders in recognizing changes in our clients – then we must have the courage and self-confidence to risk bringing it to their attention when something out of the ordinary manifests... it may save their life! Body talk equates to paying attention to details – body talk is in constant communication and we must learn to listen to the innate intelligence of what our bodies are telling us, as evidenced by the case histories shared in this book!

Thinking "out of the box" requires risk-taking steps out of our comfort zones, and sometimes out of the scope of our practice! As the aforementioned case history illustrates, it would have been a disservice to my client to allow her to leave my office without telling her she needed to see a doctor! As a healthcare practitioner, the first and foremost objective is to do no harm! While having professional experience in our chosen healing modality is important, it is our responsible choices that define us!

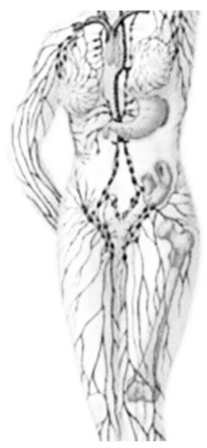

Every Woman's Fear

Sometime ago I attended a workshop where the facilitator used the term FEAR as an acronym for "false evidence appearing real." No subject matter invokes more fear in women then that of breast cancer – statistically affecting one out of five women in the U.S. Mammograms and Thermography screenings are mostly routine included in physical exams, especially for women over the age of 50. That said, these tests are also tools in proactive healthcare. This next case history speaks to every woman's plight!

A client in her early fifties called me in a perturbed voice. She had had a mammogram earlier that day and her doctor asked her to wait while he reviewed her mammogram results. Several minutes later, her doctor informed her that he found a suspicious shadow in her left breast and wanted her to have a second mammogram. She did not agree to the second mammogram and reluctantly called me and asked, "Natalie, what should I do?"

I advised her to remain positive and she should consider a lymphatic drainage massage followed by a colon hydrotherapy session.

She exclaimed, "What is lymphatic drainage?"

I explained that it is a specific kind of massage modality with a technique that assists in decongesting the lymph glands and drains pools of fluid around the lymph nodes. I told her to plan on two hours with the colon hydrotherapy to follow to facilitate moving out the toxins stimulated by the lymphatic drainage massage. She scheduled the appointment on a Tuesday and on Wednesday morning, the day after, scheduled the second mammogram. By Friday, she received the results from her doctor who said, "You know, the second mammogram showed up negative." The shadow from the first test had moved out! Obviously, the shadow seen on the first mammogram was lymph congestion. As the fluid removal was facilitated by the drainage massage, it could then be expelled through colon hydroptherapy. Her results were now "normal". My client was ecstatic, and tears of happiness replaced tears based on fears.

Lymphatic congestion may be present due to a number of factors such as lack of proper hydration because our bodies are made up 60 percent water and the rest muscles and bones. When we are not getting enough water, the body will compensate by retaining it. Lack of movement and exercise also adds to lymph congestion. Dietary concerns with foods high in sodium and acidic foods and dairy products add to the retention of fluids and the inflammation of the body as well as lymphatic overload!

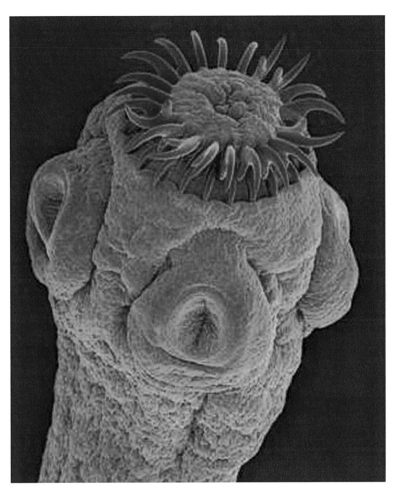

What's Eating You?

A thirty-four year old woman came to me for therapeutic massage. While having the massage, she mentioned she had multiple food allergies. I asked her what specific foods she avoided. The client responded, "I have an allergic reaction to everything I eat; it doesn't matter what! I break out in hives and begin to itch so much that I have been on a medication for 17 years called Atarax™ – it stops the itching!"

I replied, "You would benefit from a minimum series of three colon hydrotherapy sessions to detoxify and cleanse your body. I suspect it's more than just food allergies."

After her therapeutic massage, I led her to our colon hydrotherapy room and explained the procedure. She was comfortable with it and said, "I'm here; let's do this!"

The first colon hydrotherapy session began as usual with slow fills and releases to hydrate the colon and soften impacted hard stools. I suggested a light meal of salad greens and to continue hydrating with plenty of water. The amount of water I recommended is half of her body weight in ounces of water (120 lbs. equals 60 ounces of water) daily.

The second colon hydrotherapy session was the very next day – she released even more fecal matter. After the third slow fill, she released an 18" parasitic tapeworm, the head and its entire body length was expelled intact – if a section of a tapeworm breaks off, it can regenerate itself. They can grow an inch a year and release a chemical compound called Aldehydes (yes, it's like formaldehyde!) that cause a toxic reaction of hives and itching – body talk through reactions gets one's attention!

This was a tapeworm most likely from either beef or pork probably ingested from undercooked contaminated food or water contaminated by egg larvae. Another way of transmission is by auto-infestation by contaminated hands.

The client felt lighter after her colon cleansing, I then suggested an herbal parasitic cleanse be taken daily for the next 2 weeks to clear the small intestines as well as the colon. The client later called to tell me she was symptom free, no more hives or itching after she ate and was now off her medication.

BODY TALK
NEVER
LIES...

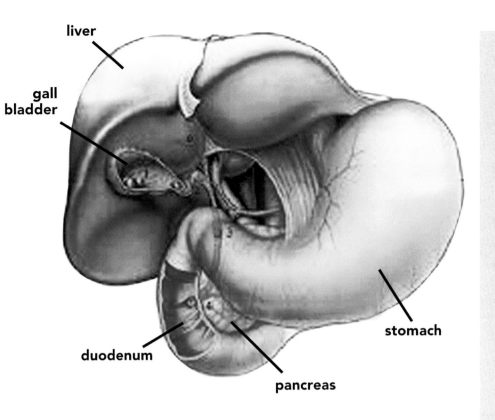

liver

gall bladder

stomach

duodenum

pancreas

Unmitigated Gall

A 24 year old woman was referred to me by her mother – a long time client. Her daughter's doctor diagnosed her as having gallstones and recommended she immediately schedule surgery for gall bladder removal. The client sought my services as she was determined to deal with this issue naturally without surgery.

I first looked at her present diet, which mainly consisted of fast-food burgers, french fries and pizza as many as 3 times a week. She preferred drinking a soda several times a day and very little water. I informed her that her present diet is highly acidic and fatty – contributing to her condition.

Gallstones are usually calcified cholesterol deposits... they can be various sizes from that like grains of sand to the size and shape of green peas or even garbanzo beans. When these stone deposits get caught in the common bile duct one can experience severe pain at the right side of the diaphragm often radiating pain to the center near the stomach.

My recommendations for her specifically included the following:

- *Have a series of six colon hydrotherapy sessions to detoxify and clear out the intestinal overload;*
- *Change and alkalize her diet – consisting of green salads with some protein;*
- *Let water be the choice of beverage and hydrate half her body weight in ounces (200 lbs. = 100 ounces of water) daily;*
- *Supplement with a full-spectrum digestive enzyme blend to support the body chemistry and assist in the breakdown and absorption of all foods – fats, proteins and carbohydrates;*
- *Add fiber and a probiotic to improve peristalsis and evacuation of her colon.*

She continued on the above support products for 60 days. Thereafter, she performed a three-day fasting and cleansing protocol along with colon hydrotherapy for each of those three days. This fast was followed by a specific holistic protocol used for a liver/gallbladder flush; each client is provided specific amounts of a natural substance made from the malic acid of apples, along with an oil and lemon juice 3 times a day over 3 days. This combination is adjusted for each individual's needs and is used to soften any stones or fatty deposits in the gallbladder.

On the fourth day, the client started to pass the softened gallstones. The client wanted a specimen of the gallstones so she brought a small jar from home to contain them. The client felt so empowered and excited about the process of ridding herself of these gallstones that she decided to take the sample to show her physician. Her doctor's response was predictable, "That's impossible. The only way you can get gallstones out is through surgery! I'll prove it to you by doing an ultra sound on you right now."

Upon performing an ultra sound, her doctor was surprised, to say the least, that there was NO evidence of gallstones! He then commented, "It must have been a misdiagnosis!"

Unmitigated
Gall

BODY TALK
NEVER
LIES...

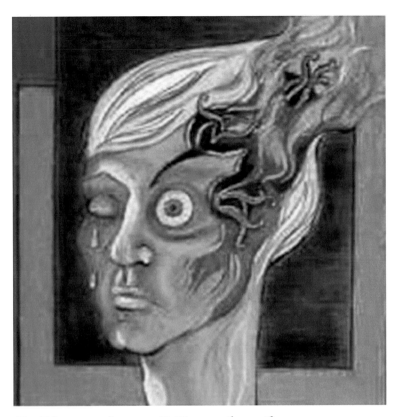

Migraine Headaches

A 35 year old female client saw me for a therapeutic massage session. She held tremendous tension in her head, neck and upper back. She revealed that she had been experiencing a migraine for the past 3 days – she was hoping the massage would ease her symptoms and rub the headache away!

Most people are unaware of the foods that can trigger headaches, particularly migraines – knowing what foods to avoid is the first step in prevention. In particular, Tyramine, a natural substance found in the breakdown of protein-based foods can trigger headaches and severe hypertension. Tyramine is found in aged cheeses, deli meats, soy sauce, organ meats, sausage, etc. Other food additives like nitrates, MSG, salt, and aspartame are food preservatives that dilate the blood vessels and cause headaches and migraines, among other health concerns like bringing excitotoxins to the brain.

I suggested to the client she consider the possibility of detoxifying her body through a series of three colon hydrotherapy sessions following the therapeutic massage. I ushered her over to the colon hydrotherapy room and showed her our equipment and explained the procedure.

I shared my experiences and methodology of why everyone should consider colonic detoxifying and cleansing to clear out the intestinal build-up of fecal impaction and putrification – preventing the recycling of toxins. I believed her migraine headaches were manifestations of these toxins recycling! Yes, weight loss is a temporary side benefit of colon hydrotherapy, but more importantly is the feeling of mental clarity, lightness and emptiness as a result of the intestinal tract reducing the body's overall toxic burden.

The client consented and proceeded to have a colon hydrotherapy session. She released so much matter during the session that she immediately felt relief from the migraine she had been battling.

Her second and third sessions proved to be even more beneficial and a healthy diet and a maintenance schedule for colon hydrotherapy have made it possible for her to now be migraine free!

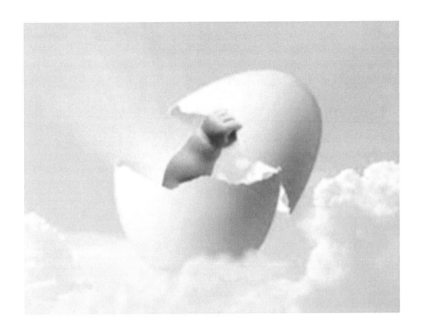

Infertility

This case history involves a 37 year old female who was referred to me with infertility issues. She had completed two in-vitro procedures with no success. Her doctor told her she needed to lose weight in order to get pregnant!

Our holistic counseling session proved beneficial in that she realized she worked far too many hours (70 hours a week) – not creating any time to have children... though she wanted them. After discussions with her focusing on the fact that we have to hold the space for what we want in our lives, often having to give up something in order to facilitate manifestation of something new in our lives, she was willing to give up her part-time job that consisted of 25 hours a week.

I focused on bringing her body into balance through nutrition, which included eating more live foods and food combining of protein with vegetables along with a green salad two times a day. Additionally, I recommended she incorporate our Body Chemistry Support System consisting of digestive enzymes, fiber, minerals and a probiotic. She also increased her hydration of water intake to ½ her body weight in ounces of water daily.

She did a series of six lymphatic massages followed by a colon hydrotherapy session as part of her detoxification protocol. She eliminated 15 pounds over the course of those weeks. Six months later I received a call from her – she had conceived and several months later gave birth to beautiful twin boys. It's amazing what our bodies can do once we provide them the natural "tools" and support the normal processes of detoxification.

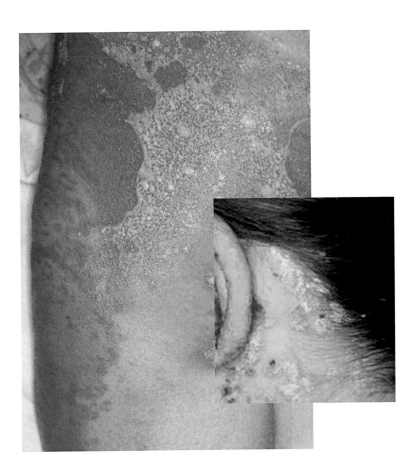

More Than Skin Deep

Though I am sharing many dramatic case histories with you, the following best exemplifies the effectiveness when a combination of treatment aspects and modalities is implemented for a serious condition, in this case, chronic psoriasis/eczema. (Explains why this story is different than others and why it is included).

The causes of Psoriasis/Eczema are not fully known, however, it is believed to be related to the body's immune system – evidenced by red scaly patches of skin, often called plaques, which build a thick layer on the skin surface. These manifestations often occur on the elbows, knees, legs, feet and hands, accompanied with intense itching and periodic flare-ups.

The body's immune response triggers, called T –Lymphocyte cells, dilate skin blood vessels in the areas around the plaque, and increase other white blood cells to merge with healthy cells. This occurrence is what forms thickening of the skin – the dead skin being unable to slough-off.

The severity of Psoriasis/eczema externally often causes loss of body image and self-consciousness. What is not seen internally is the possible causal effect known as Leaky Gut Syndrome (LGS), which causes an inflammatory response because of damage to the mucosal lining – contributing to intestinal permeability, otherwise known as autointoxication. This condition permits recycling of toxins, food, proteins and bacteria to enter into the bloodstream – manifesting as a broad range of hypersensitivity and allergic responses.

The following case history is that of a 34 year old woman with hand-sized psoriasis patches on her knees and legs – she had been suffering from this chronic condition for approximately three years. Nothing previously was effective in breaking the cycle of periodic outbreaks.

The dietary and supplemental suggestions I provided for her included:

- *address her acidic diet by avoiding all gluten, sugar, and dairy, which represents creating a more alkaline diet;*
- *eliminate the nightshades, as this genre of foods is scientifically known to induce inflammation and includes: potatoes, tomatoes, pimento, all varieties of peppers, eggplant, cayenne, and paprika;*
- *incorporate healthy greens into the diet along with limited animal proteins;*

- *increase daily hydration via water to one half of her body weight in ounces of water (130 lbs.=65 oz.).*

Because her condition warranted quickly reducing her overall body toxic load, I recommended an initial series of three colon hydrotherapy sessions over three consecutive days.

Additionally, I placed her on our body chemistry support system of supplements that included digestive enzymes, probiotics, minerals, fiber, herbal complexes and homeopathics that function as liver detoxification as well as to assist the body in purging parasitic microorganisms. These products were important in order to support her digestive system and absorption while increasing the bowel transit time along with her colon hydrotherapy sessions.

After the initial three colon therapy sessions, three days in a row, the client continued with a maintenance program over a six month period – her Psoriasis patches were completely gone after six months of colon cleansing, along with the long-standing bloating and constipation.

BODY TALK
NEVER
LIES...

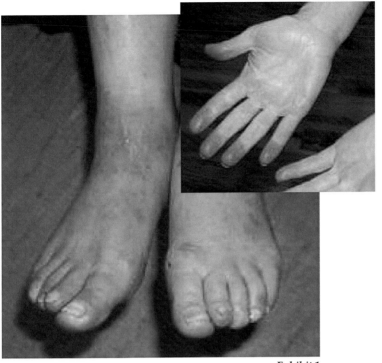

Exhibit 1

T.N.'s Story

The following is a heart-wrenching story of a young woman we'll call T.N., and her journey in dealing with a life-threatening rare disease called "Erythromelalgia" – her case being one of 13 reported cases in the world. She was referred to me by her nutritionist/homeopath, Dr. Corine Allen. Since 1996, T.N. had been receiving colon hydrotherapy to relieve constipation, toxic build-up and ameliorate the symptoms of her condition.

Erythromelalgia is a rare disease that causes severe red fevered skin and intense burning pain to the body's extremities, legs, feet, hands etc. In T.N.'s case, her legs, especially her feet, have sustained the most damage. She reports feeling as though her feet are burned from the inside out, resulting in extraordinary pain and physical trauma – see exhibit 1 for a visual representation.

In T.N.'s Own Words...

Historical Background

I've spent 14 years of my life either home bound or in hospitals. I am never pain free nor can I do anything without first considering how it will affect my condition. No one knows what causes Erythromelalgia and there is no cure. My only recourse is pain management, and a meticulously planned lifestyle.

My legs first began to ache in 1988, when I was in the eighth grade. Although I had to spend entire nights in hot water to reduce the aching, and kept a pan of cold water by my bedside to cool my feet, the doctors diagnosed my condition as "growing pains." The first clue that something was terribly wrong came during my freshman year in high school, when I suddenly found that I could not make it through a tennis match without significant pain and reddening of my feet. The redness, heat and pain started in one toe, then moved to my heels and traveled around my feet. The pain was so intense it reduced me to tears and all I could do was put them in ice water as soon as I could.

Mystified, my doctor sent me to Loma Linda University Hospital, where my condition was misdiagnosed as Raynaud's Syndrome. I was then sent to Children's Hospital in Orange, California, which also failed to achieve a correct diagnosis.

I found myself going from doctor to doctor without a correct diagnosis. By now my condition was progressing rapidly and I found it excruciating to be away from ice water. My high school freshman year ended with very little memory of anything except pain. After my freshmen year I could no longer attend school.

Finally, a dermatologist Dr. Ronald Cotliar researched and diagnosed my condition as Erythromelalgia. The recommended heavy doses of aspirin and cortisone did little

BODY TALK
NEVER
LIES...

84

good and I began to spend close to 24 hours a day in an ice water whirlpool constructed by my dad. Before long, my skin developed a Staphylococcus (Staph) infection caused by the heat of my skin and the prolonged exposure to ice water. Dr. Cotliar then proceeded to send me to UCLA Medical Center for treatment of the infection. The doctors trying to lessen my pain gave me high amounts of Morphine and Demerol, which put me in a haze but did nothing to lessen the pain and I began rubbing my feet together until my sheets were soaked in blood. Next, they gave me a saddle block, which took away the pain but left me paralyzed from the waist down. Even though I could not walk with the block at the time, it was the only relief I'd had. After three weeks my legs healed and I went home; however, with no pain control I had to begin immersing them in cold water again.

At this point with water as my only pain relief, it wasn't much longer before I found myself back at UCLA Medical Center with another staph infection. This time I was given a spinal tap numbing the nerves to my legs every three hours. They repeated this procedure so many times that each time they put the needle in my spine they would have to close the hole above as they moved down my spine so the liquid would not leak out. The once available spots on my back were exhausted from the spinal tap procedure. A constant Marcane drip was finally inserted.

My health was failing and the pain increasing. At a loss for what to do, my doctors turned to NASA. Dr. Moy from UCLA found that NASA had tried to help a girl with a similar problem and contacted them. My parents and I traveled to a NASA facility where the scientists tested me and decided to try making "cooling boots" with the same technology they used in making space suits. After I left NASA, I returned to UCLA. Dr. Nygurs from UCLA contacted Dr. George Hart at Long Beach Memorial Medical Center who agreed to

T.N.'s Story

see me. Dr. Hart was one of the pioneers of the hyperbaric oxygen chamber, which is used to heal wounds, serious burns, and more.

Meanwhile NASA was trying to get a prototype boot ready for me before my 16th birthday so I could go home with some pain control. The boots worked in keeping my feet cool. However, as they were a prototype, all the bugs were not out of the design yet. The skin on my legs was fragile and the boots caused condensation between the inside lining and my skin. My legs and feet developed Trench Foot from the moisture. When I saw Dr. Hart, he wasn't sure he could even save my legs – I had ulcers and open sores on 80% of my skin below my knees. I spent the next six weeks in the hospital in wound care where it was also discovered I had developed Spinal Meningitis as a result of the UCLA spinal taps. After six weeks in the hospital, I was then treated on an outpatient basis for the next 4 months – we'd arrive at 7 a.m. and depart around 10 p.m. seven days a week, staying in our motor home in the parking lot of the hospital. When we arrived in the morning, I had wound care followed by hyperbaric oxygen treatment and then repeated this process in the evening. The good news, Dr. Hart saved my legs. The bad news, still no pain control. I kept my feet out of the water as much as possible. In a desperate attempt to keep my feet cool without using water, my Mom and I drove around late at night with my feet out the window of the car – the only way I got some relief and much needed sleep.

All this time I was in survival mode with what seemed like no days and nights – only time filled with pain. I was bed-ridden in a hospital bed setup in our family room. My parents kept the room very cold to help my feet. I withdrew inside myself to garner the strength to simply survive.

For five years I never left the house, except to go to the hospital. One of my few good memories of those days was getting to go to one of my brother's high school football games. We were able to park right down on the end of the field and I watched from the motor home. He was the quarterback and it was the only game my Mom and I got to see that year. His school was great to let us do this because at that time I was connected to IVs.

Schooling was very difficult for me. Not only did the constant pain and doctor appointments make concentrating on studies very difficult, but also made class schedules nearly impossible. My parents withdrew me from high school after my freshman year. I was home schooled for the next three years by a teacher named Mr. Cole. Through constant support and dedication, Mr. Cole helped me to graduate on time with my class in 1993. At the time of graduation I could not walk on my own – my brother carried me to the platform to receive my diploma.

Shortly after graduation, we headed in our motor home for the Mayo Clinic in Rochester, Minnesota. Throughout the trip I kept my legs wrapped in gauze so I could spray them with water while a fan blew air on them. Dr. Rooke at Mayo took an interest in the disease and me. Much to his credit, he wanted to do more research on Erythromelalgia but it is very hard to get funding for a disease that affects only a small group of people.

When we returned home from the Mayo Clinic we began a new program through Long Beach Memorial Medical Center. I was the youngest person to receive a Medtronic Pain Pump. The pain pump, surgically inserted into my abdomen, administered a combination of drugs through an epidural that continually numbs specific nerves, reducing my pain. The pump was not without problems. First, it has to be replaced every few years requiring intensive surgery and a huge cost. Second, the pump needs to be refilled with the drugs once a week by a doctor using a syringe to access a

T.N.'s Story

pump port located underneath the skin of my stomach–a process that is not without risks. A doctor once missed the port and injected the drugs into my system causing me to go into shock. Even with its risks, the pump was the first thing that had allowed me to try and manage pain and have some quality of life again.

While the pain was becoming manageable, the heat continued to affect my legs physically causing burns and sores. My legs are medically defined as an "open wound." I eventually discovered a homeopathic doctor whose treatment helped me improve their condition through homeopathic remedies and acupuncture.

I continue to make annual trips to the Mayo Clinic. During one of these trips I underwent a therapy called Phoresis to clean my blood and was once again able to walk, although unable to walk any distance. My dad suggested I try riding a bike. At first I rode only short distances, but over time I increased my ability and found that riding improved my circulation and helped improve my condition.

Another factor that assists improving my condition is elevation. We found that putting me at a high cool elevation, such as that of Breckenridge, Colorado at 9,600 feet, has a wonderful effect on my condition. When at that altitude, I'm able to use much less medication and stay far more comfortable than at home in California. Now, we travel to Colorado each summer to spend time away from the California heat. Unfortunately, the cold winters of Colorado are as bad for my feet as the California summers, so I cannot stay there year round.

Each of the specific factors previously outlined enables me to maintain a daily schedule and gives me a sense of independence and control over my life – something I have never had. When I go out of the house, I have to ensure that I am properly prepared. I must be stable and have my pain under control – my fans, computer, medications and cell phone go with me everywhere. My fans help to cool my feet and legs and my computer enables me to adjust my medication. I have to make sure someone is available to pick me up if my condition flares up, and I cannot drive far because I need to be close enough that someone can reach me quickly. Additionally, my workout needs to be completed for the day. I workout every morning, ride my bike 20-30 miles in the evening and 10 minutes on the stationary bike at night. These workouts have helped me to reduce the amount of pain medication I need. In short, it is a combination of all aspects of my routine that allow me to function.

Although I was able to get my driver's license, the level that my feet rest on the pedals is so far below my heart it severely increases the blood flow to my feet and also increases my pain. This increase in pain is dangerous because it causes me to focus on my legs and not my driving. At the same time, I have a hard time sitting still because I spent so many years in bed and I don't want to miss any more of my life.

I live in constant fear that the pain will return, so I carry out my daily regimen with diligence – the reality, pain is just a malfunction away. When the pump fails for any reason all the pain returns with vengeance! This is a true reality for me, but I am determined to live as normal a life as possible. We with rare diseases have a hard time constantly explaining to others what our condition is, why we behave the way we do, and why it consumes so much of our lives. But I live in hope and gratitude…

Hope that each day I will be able to do things I need to manage my pain...

... that one day a treatment and/or cure for Erythromelalgia will be found.

Grateful that I am able to get out of bed and live my life...

... to my parents and all they do to help me live with my condition.

Sincerely, T. N.
October 30, 2011

Written permission granted by client to recall her story in her own words.

T.N.'s Story

T.N.'s Testinmonial

I really didn't know what a colonic was but we made an appointment with Natalie Davis. My first impression of Natalie was the most important and that impression turned out to be correct – she was non-threatening, caring, and encouraging...all at the same time. In her extremely professional persona, she explained to me and my parents what to expect at every aspect of the therapy and the way this procedure was important for my body and quality of life, especially for such a serious medical condition.

I always step carefully into new things, especially after what my family and I have been through. Having to go over my entire health history repeatedly from doctor to doctor and therapist to therapist becomes very laboring, to say the least.

In dealing with Natalie, something about her and her quiet knowingness and caring was very different – she actually listened to what I said, which I have found out is quite rare in health professionals these days.
It wasn't simply a robotic-type of routine she was going through; she was computing everything I said in her head.

There are many things that I went through that I have not mentioned in this brief testimonial or my story– staph infections, operations, etc. And unlike other patients, I have to have a fan on my feet and legs the entire time Natalie works on me plus I cannot lay on my stomach because I have a internal pump implant in my stomach. Nothing bothered Natalie; she just smiled making no qualms about any special accommodations, which always puts me at complete ease while in her care.

I not only have this rare condition severely in my feet and legs but, to a lesser degree, I also have it in my hands

and they can become very uncomfortable, red and hot. One of the things I noticed almost right away after my colon hydrotherapy is that my hands would no longer be red and painful.

Colon hydrotherapy does not cure my EM condition, however, it really helps control the effect this terribly painful and life-limiting condition has on my body. The medications I have to take, and those the doctors have tried over the years, built up in my body and I could not get rid of the toxic overload. Colon hydrotherapy enables my body to eliminate these toxins faster and in a healthy way – facilitating a huge break away from this continued bombardment of chemicals and it also lessens the outbreaks of EM.

Colon hydrotherapy has allowed my body to become healthier. If the body cannot get rid of the toxic over load, those toxins add to the damage already being done by the disease itself. Chemicals are chemicals, whether they come from prescription or over-the-counter medications, environmental poisons, food laced with chemicals – preservatives – flavor enhancers – chemical sweeteners, etc. – colon hydrotherapy helps in reducing the overall toxic load!

When I first started the therapy, I had to see Natalie at least once a week. As I improved, we were able to find an acceptable maintenance program for my condition.

Natalie has become a dear person to me from the first encounter in her office. She's always caring, professional, and knowledgeable; which is really important when under going any procedure, especially one as intimate as colon hydrotherapy. Over the years she has encouraged me by always infusing that extra boost of confidence when a difficult situation arises – so important to any patient, especially those with chronic and challenging health conditions like mine.

T.N.'s Testimonial

91

BODY TALK
NEVER
LIES...

Afterword...

My sincere desire for all of you is that the essence of the client and case histories I've shared will assist both the health professional and client in sculpting away regressed traumas and memories to reveal their true essence.

Colon hydrotherapy and Transformational Bodywork (TBW) encompass the true spirit of practitioner and client working together to explore the art of personal disarmament and conscious creative living.

The TBW approach to balanced and joyous living is aimed at awareness itself though it works deeply with the physical body. In neutralizing the reactivity of the neuro-emotional musculature a flow state emerges that reveals what the individual truly embodies. This awareness leads to the resolution of unhealed wounds and to the release of creative life force. In practical ways, faith, compassion and forgiveness meet unconscious cellular memories – bringing the healing wisdom of the breath out of the shadows. Thus, a space opens where gratitude, humor and security can exist in a world of impermanence.

The focus of *Body Talk NEVER Lies* is to shine upon the causal place in the armament of the physical body where unconscious beliefs, repressed memory and charged unresolved emotional experience co-exist. The reactivity and tension of this armament are accessed through the breath, subtle energy fields and deep tissue manipulation of the musculature – allowing trapped creative energy and unhealed wounds to be revealed and healed.

To Your Health,

Natalie